The Bilingual Encounter with Aphasia

THE PATTERNS OF REHABILITATION OF APHASIA FOR BILINGUAL HISPANICS

by

AF870899

Ferdinand Garcia

Dual Masters of Science and Education
in Bilingual Education in the Graduate School of Education in The City College of New York

ISHI PRESS
INTERNATIONAL

The Bilingual Encounter with Aphasia

THE PATTERNS OF REHABILITATION OF APHASIA FOR BILINGUAL HISPANICS

by
Ferdinand Garcia

Dual Masters of Science and Education
in Bilingual Education in the
Graduate School of Education in
The City College of New York

Published November 15, 2010
by Ishi Press in New York and Tokyo

ferdinandgrc@yahoo.com

ISBN 4-87187-715-9
978-4-87187-715-2

Ishi Press International
1664 Davidson Avenue, Suite 1B
Bronx NY 10453-7877
USA

1-917-507-7226

Printed in the United States of America

Dedication

This research / book is dedicated in memory of my mother Eulalia Flores Garcia born in Cidra Puerto Rico, February 12, 1921 - Died October 8 , 2009, who suffered a stroke and was diagnosed with Broker's Aphasia.

Acknowledgments

I would like to thank my brother David Garcia who dedicated twenty four seven of his time for seven years caring for our mother. I would also like to thank my oldest sister sally and her family, and my youngest sister Evelyn and her family.

I also wish to thank George Gracia, who assisted in this research project.

TABLE OF CONTENTS

CHAPTER I

THE PROBLEM

This research is focused on "***Aphasia***", a condition caused by neurological damage. The search is to find how psychologists, neurologists, and speech pathologists can help bilingual Hispanics with aphasia when the ability to understand language and to translate thoughts into words is impaired.

Introduction

Aphasia is a condition caused by neurological damage or disease to the brain, which affects a person's ability to communicate. "The use of speech to communicate is unique to humans. When speech is impaired or absent, the impact on the person and his/her family is profound. One of the most heartbreaking and devastating disabilities is aphasia. Most people have not heard about aphasia, nor do they know the term until someone in their family or a friend acquires aphasia." (National Aphasia Association Fact Sheet, 2001.)

Patients with speech problems gave early researchers the first clues about how the brain is involved with language. The loss of the ability to speak is called "aphasia." The ancient Greeks noticed that brain damage could cause aphasia.

Pierre Paul Broca, (1824-1880) was born in **Bordeaux, France**. He studied mathematics and physical science, and trained as a pathologist, anatomist, and surgeon. Broca made significant contributions to other fields most notably to anthropology. The discovery in **1856** of **Neanderthal man** drew Broca into anthropology. Broca is best known for his role in the discovery of specialized functions in different areas of the brain. His post-mortem analysis of patients, who lost the ability to speak, associated damage to specific areas of the brain. In particular, the front of the brain's left side. Human speech requires codifying thought and transmitting it in patterned strings of sound. The area of the brain isolated by Broca sends the code to another part of the brain that controls the muscles of the face, jaw, tongue, palate, and larynx, setting the speech apparatus in motion. This area and a companion area that controls the understanding of language, known as Wernicke's area, are detectable in early fossil skulls of the genus Homo. The brain of Homo was evolving toward the use of language, although the vocal chamber was still inadequate to articulate speech. Broca discovered one piece in the puzzle of human communication and speech, which permits the transmission of culture. Equally important, Broca contributed to the development of physical anthropology, one of the four subfields of anthropology. Craniology, the scientific measurement of the skull, was a major focus of physical anthropology during this period. Broca furthered these studies by inventing at least twenty-seven instruments for making measurements of the human body, and by developing standardized techniques of measurement. ***The Gale Encyclopedia of Psychology, Gale Encyclopedia of Psychology, 2nd ed. Gale Group, (2001)***.

Broca and Wernicke's aphasias involve language functioning. Patients with speech problems gave early researchers the first clues about how the brain is involved with language. In 1861, Paul Broca described a patient who could say only one word "***Tan***". For this reason, Broca called this patient "**Tan**". When Tan died, Broca examined his brain and found that there was damage to part of the left frontal cortex, which is the outer layer or gray matter of the brain. This part of the brain has come to be known as Broca's Area. Broca's speech is often telegraphic, communicating using short words, less than four words, and grammatical. It sounds a lot like the way Tan talked, he did not use function words like conjunctions, articles, or prepositions. However auditory comprehension is usually much better than speech. Thus, never assume that just because a person can't express himself and is paralyzed that he can't understand you.

Carl Wernicke, 1848-1905, was a German neurologist born in Tarnovitz, Poland, but his family moved to Germany where he received all his education. His initial Interest was in psychiatry; he studied anatomy, and neuropathology later. He published a small volume on aphasia, which vaulted him into international fame. In it was precise pathoanatomic analysis paralleling the clinical picture. He is best known for his work on sensory aphasia in which the affected individual speaks words fluently but without meaningful content.

http://www.uic.edu/depts/mcne/founders/page0101.html

Wernicke discovered a lesion in the brain resulting in damage to the upper rear part of the left temporal lobe. Wernicke is important for his work in relating nerve diseases to specific areas of the brain. The last two decades of his life were spent as professor of neurology and psychiatry first at Breslau and then at Halle, Germany. Wernicke belonged to a 19th century school of German neuropsychiatry that made no distinction between disorders of the mind and disorders of the brain. He is best known for his studies of aphasia, according to Merriam-Webster, Inc.

http://www.fasthealth.com/dictionary/w/Wernicke_aphasia.php.

In contrast to Broca's area, the speech of Wernicke's aphasics is fluent and often rapid, but with relatively empty content and many neologisms (invented words) and word substitutions. Knowing information about traumatic brain injury should help speech pathologists understand how aphasia affects a person's ability to manipulate speech, sounds, vocabulary, grammar and meaning. Broca's aphasia, which is characterized by slow and labored speech with prepositions and articles missing, for example, "I went store," does not affect comprehension of written and spoken language.

Statement of the Problem

"Damage to Broca's area results in marked problems with language fluency, with shortened sentences, impaired flow of speech, poor control of rhythm and intonation (known as prosody); and a telegraphic style, with missing inflections and function words." Information taken from an online article on Language Disorder from the **Gale Encyclopedia of Psychology, 2nd ed. Gale Group, (2001)**.

There are limited studies done among bilingual Hispanics patients with aphasia. According to therapists in urban rehabilitation facilities, treatment for all patients with aphasia are conducted in English only. The speech pathologists at the treatment facilities were not proficient in speaking Spanish, therefore, bilingual Hispanic patients could not be provided with adequate therapy. Knowing information about traumatic brain injury should help speech pathologists understand how aphasia affects a person's ability to manipulate speech, sounds, vocabulary, grammar and meaning. Facilities that do not have therapists who understand the patient's language hinder the rehabilitation process for bilingual Hispanic patients.

Research Questions

In order to contribute to a more comprehensive understanding of aphasia the following research questions were considered:

What rehabilitation and patterns were helpful?

How many and what type of battery tests were conducted?

What type of treatment was provided?

Where was the therapy given?

Definitions of Terms

Aphasia

"Is condition characterized by either partial or total loss of the ability to communicate verbally or using written words. A person with aphasia may have difficulty speaking, reading, writing, recognizing the names of objects, or understanding what other people have said. The term aphasia is caused by a brain injury, as may occur during a traumatic accident, or when the brain is deprived of oxygen during a stroke. A brain tumor, a disease such as Alzheimer's, or an infection, like encephalitis, may also cause aphasia. Aphasia may be temporary or permanent. Aphasia does not include speech impediments caused by loss of muscle control."(p 2,5). Taken from Barrett K. (2001). Aphasia. Gale Encyclopedia of Medicine.

Broca's Aphasia

Is a form of aphasia in which speech output is severely reduced and is limited mainly to short utterances, of less than four words. Vocabulary access is limited in persons with Broca's aphasia, and their formation of sounds is often laborious and clumsy. The person may understand speech relatively well and be able to read, but be limited in writing. Broca's aphasia is often referred to as a 'non fluent aphasia' because of the halting and effortful quality of speech. Cf. **Merriam-Webster, Inc.**

Conduction Aphasia

A fluent aphasia, usually caused by lesion that interrupt the actuate fasciculus's the primary nerve pathway connecting Wernicke's and Broca's areas. Patients with conduction aphasia usually have good language comprehension, because the primary auditory cortex and auditory association area (Wernicke's area) are intact. However, because the connections between the auditory and language areas and the area for planning and executing speech (and writing) have been impaired, conduction regions, that is, overlapping and interconnected neural networks widely distributed throughout the brain, carrying out their specific neural functions both sequentially and in parallel. The concept of parallel distributed processing (POP), popular in contemporary cognitive science, provides a useful metaphor for the understanding of higher cortical functions in humans. The simplest language task depends on a complex interaction of the reticular activating system, subcortical nuclear structures, right hemisphere, subcortical white matter, and left-hemispheric "zone of language."

Wernicke's Aphasia

Is another form of aphasia. Wernicke's aphasics have fluent spontaneous speech where there are frequent paraphasias and/or neologisms (new words), and speech may be described as jargon. Word comprehension is poor, and repetition is also disturbed.

http://www.uic.edu/depts/mcne/founders/page0101

The following definitions of terms according to the chapter on Neuroanatomy of Language from the Manual of Aphasia Therapy **(Helm-Estabrooks 1983)**.

Subcortical Structures and Brainstem

Subcortical Structures

Corpus callosum

Connects right with left cerebral hemispheres anterior commissure accessory to corpus callosumfornix - connects midbrain and hypothalamus to hippocampus:

hippocampus - involved in memory

basal nuclei (ganglia) - modulates muscle tone

caudate nucleus - largest of the basal nuclei

pineal gland - involved in circadian rhythms using melatonin

thalamus - filter and select sensory information

lateral geniculate nuclei - for vision, cn II medial

geniculate nuclei - for hearing, cn XIII

intermediate mass - connection between right and left thalamus.

Brain Stem

Medulla oblongata

Is the continuation of the spinal cord through the base of the skull. This portion of the brain stem contains nuclei for the cranial nerves responsible for movements of the tongue, orpharynx, larynx, and diaphragm.

Pons

Is continuous with the medulla, and the midbrain is continuous with the pons. These segments of the brain contain cranial nerve nuclei for eye movements, facial expression, facial sensation, and hearing.

Cranial nerves - 1 thru XII as follows:

Olfactory nerve (I) - special sensory, smell

Optic nerve (II) - special sensory, vision

Oculomotor nerve (Ill) - motor, eye movement

Trochlear nerve (IV) - motor, eye movement (superior oblique muscle)

Trigeminal nerve (V) - mixed sensory and motor; face, mouth, mastication

Abducens nerve (VI) - motor, eye movement (lateral rectus)

Facial nerve (VII) - mixed sensory and motor; anterior 2/3 tongue, facial expression

Vestibulocochlear nerve (VIII) - special sensory, balance and hearing

Glossopharyngeal nerve (IX) - mixed sensory and motor; posterior 1/3 tongue, carotid arteries, swallowing

Vagus nerve (X) - mixed sensory and motor; visceral organs

Spinal accessory (XI)- motor, neck

Hypoglossal nerve (XII) - motor, tongue movements.

The following definitions of terms are from the ***Webster's Ninth New Collegiate Dictionary (1991).***

Cortex

Relating to or consisting of cortex. The outer or superficial part of an organ or body structure. The outer layer of gray matter of the cerebrum and cerebellum.

Lesions

Abnormal change in the structure of an organ or part due to injury or disease.

Hemiparesis

Half side, paresis slight or partial paralysis.

Infract

Break off.

Ischemia

Localized tissue anemia due to obstruction of the inflow of arterial blood.

Caudate

Have a tail or a tail like appendage.

Sensory

Of or relating to sensation or to the senses. Conveying nerve impulses from the sense organs to the nerve centers.

Receptive

A sensory end organ; fit to receive and transmit stimuli. **Posterior**

Behind.

Motor Motion.

Relating to or being a nerve or nerve fiber that passes from the central nervous system or ganglion toward or to a muscle and conducts an impulse that causes movement.

CHAPTER II

REVIEW OF THE RELATED LITERATURE

Introduction

Aphasia is a condition caused by neurological damage or disease to the brain, which affects a person's ability to communicate. "The use of speech to communicate is unique to humans. When speech is impaired or absent, the impact on the person and his/her family is profound. One of the most heartbreaking and devastating disabilities is aphasia. Most people have not heard about aphasia, nor do they know the term until someone in their family or a friend acquires aphasia. (**National Aphasia Association Fact Sheet, (2001**).

The definition of aphasia taken from the ***Gale Encyclopedia of Medicine*** `is condition characterized by either partial or total loss of the ability to communicate verbally or using written words. A person with aphasia may have difficulty speaking, reading, writing, recognizing the names of objects, or understanding what other people have said. Aphasia is caused by a brain injury, as may occur during a traumatic accident, or when the brain is deprived of oxygen during a stroke. A brain tumor, a disease such as Alzheimer's, or an infection, like encephalitis, may also cause aphasia. Aphasia may be temporary or permanent. Aphasia does not include speech impediments caused by loss of muscle control. (p 2-5)

This research will focus on how neurologists and speech pathologists can help bilingual Hispanics with aphasia when the ability to understand language and to translate thoughts into words is impaired as a result of a traumatic brain injury. In order to contribute to a more comprehensive understanding of aphasia the following research questions will be considered:

What rehabilitation and patterns were helpful?

How many and what type of battery tests were conducted?

What type of treatment was provided?

Where was the therapy given?

Patients with speech problems gave early researchers the first clues about how the brain is involved with language. The loss of the ability to speak is called "aphasia." The ancient Greeks noticed that brain damage could cause aphasia. A quarter century later in 1861, Paul Broca described a patient who could say one word "***Tan***". For this reason, Broca called this patient "Tan." When Tan died, Broca examined his brain and found that there was damage to part of the left frontal cortex. This part of the brain has come to be known as Broca's Area.") See Figure 1

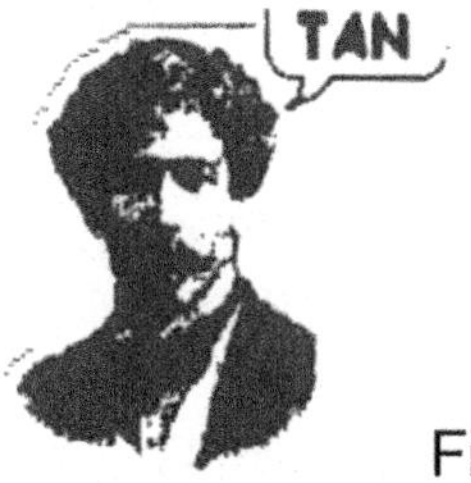

Figure 1

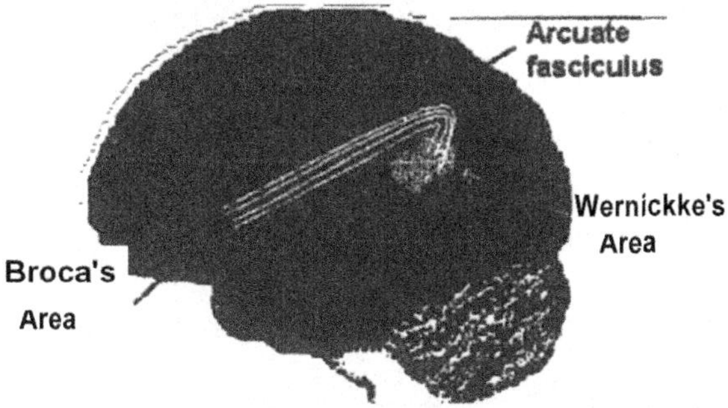

Left frontal cortex. Also known as Broca's Area.

Located in the posterior part of the temporal lobe.

Fig. 2. Frontal Lobe

Fig. 2. Frontal Lobe

An article online by Sherny T. Gilesche, "Aphasia". Archived file at **http://www.imssf.org/aphasia/htm**, states, "Damage to the brain affects how an individual language comprehension is processed. As a result of the injury, the damage can affect the frontal lobe area of the left hemisphere of the brain known as Broca's area of Aphasia (also called Motor, Expressive, or Anterior Aphasia): Broca's' aphasia is usually seen following damage to the posterior inferior frontal lobe, obviously called Broca's'area. Hemiplegia (paralysis of one side of the body) or hemiphareis (weakness of one side of the body) usually accompanies Broca's aphasia. See figure 2.

For right-handers the paralysis or paresis is almost always on the right, because lesions causing aphasia are almost always left-hemisphere lesions, and motor control is contra lateral. Symptoms: Speech is nonfluent, labored, and halting. Intonation and stress patterns are deficient, and misarticulating is prominent.

Broca's speech is often telegraphic and agrammatical. (Not meaning to be rude here, but it sounds a lot like the way Tan talks; no function words like conjunctions, articles, or prepositions.) but, their auditory comprehension is usually much better than their speech! (So never assume that just because a person can't express himself and is paralyzed that he can't understand you!)

Paul Broca (born 1824 – died 1880) was a French doctor who specialized in the functioning of the left and right side of the brain. **Carl Wernicke** (1848-1905) was a German neurologist who discovered a lesion in the brain resulting in damage to the upper rear part of the left temporal lobe. Broca and Wernicke's aphasias involve language functioning. Patients with speech problems gave early researchers the first clues about how the brain is involved with language. The loss of the ability to speak is called "aphasia." In 1876, Carl Wemicke found that damage to a different part of the brain also caused language problems. This area of the brain ('Wemicke's Area") was further back and lower in the brain compared to Broca's area. In fact, Wemicke's area is in the posterior part of the temporal lobe. Broca's area and Wemicke's area are connected by a bund of nerve fibers called the actuate fasciculus's. Damage to the actuate fasciculus's causes a disorder called conduction aphasia. People with conduction aphasia can understand language, but their speech does not make sense and they cannot repeat words.

Information taken from an online article on Language Disorder from the Gale Encyclopedia of Psychology states, "Damage to Broca's area results in marked problems with language fluency, with shortened sentences, impaired flow of speech, poor control of rhythm and intonation (known as prosody); and a telegraphic style, with missing inflections and function words. In contrast, the speech of Wernicke's aphasics is fluent and often rapid, but with relatively empty content and many neologisms (invented words) and word substitutions. Knowing information about traumatic brain injury should help Speech pathologists understand how aphasia affects a person's ability to manipulate speech, sounds, vocabulary, grammar and meaning. Broca's aphasia, which is characterized by slow and labored speech with prepositions and articles missing, for example, "I went store," which does not affect comprehension of written and spoken language. There are many classifications of aphasia, such as Global, which is widespread damage to the dominant cerebral hemisphere, either right or left, and is almost a total loss of the ability for speech, comprehension, reading and writing. Dysphasia describes a general loss of language use. Dysgraphia deals with problems associated with writing, and agraphia is the complete inability to write. (According to an article on **Aphasia, Gale Encyclopedia of Childhood and Adolescence**.)

Language disorder by Jill De Villers, Ph.D. online **Problem with any function of language and communication**.

According to an article on **Aphasia, Gale Encyclopedia of Medicine**, stroke is the most common cause of aphasia in the United States. Approximately 500,000 individuals suffer strokes each year and 20 percent of these individuals develop some type of Aphasia. Other causes of brain damage include head injuries, brain tumors, and infections. Some individuals can recover quickly within a few days or it can take years especially for individuals with traumatic brain injury.

A person experiences memory loss, especially after a traumatic brain injury. It is usually sudden and it can be temporary or permanent. Memory loss that is age-related such as Alzheimer's disease occurs gradually and is usually permanent. In short-term memory loss, a person cannot remember daily events or remember what happened within the past few minutes, but can remember events from their childhood. In long-term memory loss, a person is unable to remember events from the past. Consequently, after a severe brain injury a person can lose their memory and consciousness, and then fully recover. The following review will look at head injuries after a motor vehicle accident.

According to the article by **Kreutzer and Witol (1996)** pps. 8, 10,11 "Supported Employment as an Option for Return to Competitive Employment," head injuries usually affect young men. Sixty percent of traumatic brain injury (TBI) victims are males under the age of 35. It is estimated that motor vehicle accidents resulted in approximately 200 TBI per 100,000 populations. This is a group of individuals who have impaired cognition in the area of short-term memory, processing, planning, judgment and sequencing. They also exhibit problems in psychosocial behavior, which accounts for insubordinate and disruptive social behaviors at work, depression, seizures, educational abilities, and physical competence.

Head injuries can be classified as penetrating or closed head injuries. Penetrating head injuries tend to be more localized damage and more predictable and discrete disabilities than closed head injuries. A bullet lacerates the scalp, fractures the skull and rips the soft tissue, killing nerve cells in the process. A closed head injury is caused by the head hitting another surface, such as a car windshield, which results in the brain smashing against the inner surface of the skull. Closed brain injuries result in many disabilities requiring post-trauma recovery from a few months to several years. "A Glasgow Coma Scale (GCS) is a 15 point standardized instrument for assessing overall neurological response or outcome after a head injury. Many patients remain in a coma from one to nine months. About 5 percent of all head injuries are defined as severe head injuries." These individuals are likely to have brain stem damage resulting in severe permanent physical disabilities such as paralysis, weakness, plasticity, and tremors. Speech is often affected and the individual can spend a year or more in a hospital rehabilitation setting. Progress is slow and can take many years before returning to work and it is usually in a reduced capacity. The range of deficits are many including an executive deficit which sets brain injured victims apart from other disabled individuals. For instance, individuals who become disabled may have physical disabilities to their bodies, but their brain is intact. An executive deficit deals with problems in goal formation, processing, executing plans, self-monitoring, awareness of others, and ability to anticipate.

These are abilities that help an individual stay in a job. (According to the article, "***Employers' attitude toward hiring persons with disabilities and vocational***

rehabilitation services.")

In a study reported in the article, "***Supported Employment as an Option for Return to Competitive Employment***," Kreutzer and Witol (1996), five clients were selected between the ages 20 to 37 and referred to a supported employment program in Virginia. Parents, private and public rehabilitation counselors, physicians, local hospitals, and insurance companies referred them. All were injured in motor vehicle accidents. It is important to know the level of functioning prior to the head injury. Therefore, data collected from family members revealed all experienced behavioral problems before being injured including substance abuse. One graduated from college and two graduated from high school. Further neuropsychological evaluations assists the job coach to apply existing skills by understanding specific cognitive dysfunctions and limitations for new learning and problem solving. Thus, job training and placement considers past experiences, and is based on client interest, such as going to work and keeping a job, job compatibility, job availability, transportation services, and family support.

The job coach follows up with the patient for about 18 months. However, persons with TBI often require placement into other jobs as compared to other disabled adults due to consistently changing vocational aspirations and behaviors. Swearing and angry outbursts on the job and other problems also emerge away from the job; for instance, excessive drinking that can impair a person's ability to continue on the job.

Re-educating and providing a person with the necessary available resources after a head injury have a far-reaching impact to let that person know he/she can work. It also proves that TBI does not mean handicap, and that self-sufficiency is possible.

Grosjean (1982) says educators/speech pathologist have to start teaching students from the beginning as if from the age of zero for the student to learn the target language whether it is in English or Spanish and this is where Bilingualism is included. It is believed no matter the age of the person the methods to teach a person with aphasia is the same for any learning disability. Learning to speak is in stages. Language variety and the formulated order begin from the age of zero to pre-adulthood. Krashen (1996), a theorist, says the hypothesis of natural acquisition order is that everyone develops sounds in the same order. The person begins by first developing consonants. The sounds of the consonants forming the two lips sounds that are: m for mama, b for bottle, and p for papa. Then the vowel sounds are the second step of acquiring language. Teaching the student English grammar noun and verb endings are the two areas under the ending of sound. Nouns, which are taught in the beginning, such as: ***s*** plural, ***books***; and ***s*** possessive, ***Mary's*** books. The second area under sound ending is: ***ing***, which is an infinitive ending in a verb within the language of English and Spanish. In English, we recognize i***ng*** as an infinitive ending in a verb. In Spanish, ***ando - caminando***, (walking). We also recognize ***ed*** as a past participle and ***ed*** in past tense and we also recognize ***s*** as a verb ending. These are steps used to re-teach pronunciation to people with aphasia. This language acquisition order registers the process of learning the correct pronunciation as the individual with aphasia continues to learn by practice and repetition.

However, to begin the teaching process, the first step should be to identify and diagnose the learning disability by knowing the person's medical and personal history. It also helps to identify how well a person's motor skills are in order to determine the ability to perform certain tasks. After assessing the patient's weaknesses and strengths, an individualized plan is developed noting what the patient can or cannot do. For instance, leaving out words, fails to hear sounds, difficulty manipulating thoughts into words.

Many of the special education strategies for a person with a learning disability are basically good teaching techniques. For example, telling a patient in advance what they will learn, the benefits of certain methods, using visual aids, providing listening, speaking, reading written assignments, and giving oral and written instructions to help the patient focus and remember key parts. With the advancement in technology and widespread use of computers at school and home, therapist can expand and utilize alternative teaching tools. Sounds can be repeated, and visual aids can help the process to manipulate thoughts and sounds into meaningful words.

Adjustments to Disability

Along with re-education the patient with aphasia, psychologists, therapists and the family must help the patient to accept that they have to adjust to a different quality of life and ultimate functional abilities. According to **Kreutzer and Witol (1996)**, person who has sustained a severe brain injury must begin by developing a new sense of self. A brain injury dramatically changes a person's life and their family life. Making adjustments means that a person recognizes that they cannot go back to the way they were. They need to move forward by taking steps to adjust to the new limitations resulting from the brain injury as they develop their new sense of self-awareness.

Family support is extremely important during the various stages of recovery. For example, a friend's son at age 32, worked as an engineer in the Texas oil fields. One evening while driving home from work he hit a tractor-trailer's side head-on and sustained a severe brain injury. He was in a coma for about two months and afterwards required extensive rehabilitation. Eventually his mother relocated him from Texas to New Jersey. She moved to a two? bedroom apartment to accommodate her son and care for him until he died four years later from recurring brain infections. The readjustment and caring at times was difficult as his speech was impaired, he was forgetful, often very frustrated at the slow progress, had angry outbursts, and cursed.

Building self-esteem and encouragement is part of the recovery process. The family reinforces behaviors they would like to see, and ignoring behaviors that should be decreased. Quite often restructuring the living environment, such as planning meal schedules and even rest periods. It is important that the family member(s) help to redirect the person rather than challenge the person when it takes longer to do even daily routine tasks. (***Kreutzer et al.***)

Evaluation

An evaluation of the patient's progress that includes the home life and treatment care must occur throughout the patient's recovery. The therapists need to evaluate how well he/she is doing and also evaluate the stages of learning development of the patient. The evaluation process should include the patient, the family members and the therapist's performance as well as obtaining feedback from agencies providing care for the patient. Questionnaires can be used to survey family members and make telephone calls to gain insight on how the person is doing at home and the impact on the family life. If the person is working, find out how they are functioning on the job. The therapist can design an evaluation tool to ask the patient for feedback about areas for improvement and what the patient would like to see changed or improved on.

Cultural Diversity

As the TBI works towards re-healing, being culturally sensitive is extremely important as well as being aware of ethnic and religious differences as traumatic brain injury affects everyone, all cultures. These individuals come from all lifestyles and occupations, and they can be rich or poor. For instance, supported employment helps individuals with severe disabilities to become productive members of society by recognizing and providing access to employment opportunities. It took a long time for a male Hispanic friend to seek help from supported employment. The staff working with this individual had to respect the fact that he was very proud and not be overbearing. Further, economically, TBI does not discriminate. The Brain Injury Association has helped families with little or no money to assist in caring for the person with TBI, and a family with all their money cannot do anything to help their family member come out of a coma. (**Kreutzer et al. (1996)**)

Neurogenic Communication Disorders in Bilingual Adults: Bilingual Aphasia: A Case Study. Reyes, B.A., Peterson, C.S. (1997).

According to the U.S. Bureau of Census (1990), there are at a minimum 25 million people in this country who are bilingual. Within the next 10 years, Hispanics will account for the largest minority in the U.S. 65 percent are bilingual, the rest Spanish speaking. Clearly, speech-language pathologists can expect to be faced with an increasing number of bilingual patients with aphasia as a result from a brain injury, stroke or disease as the population ages.

A case study by **Reyes, B.A., Peterson, C.S. (1997)** is about a bilingual Hispanic patient with aphasia. Specifically, the case study focuses on bilingualism and code switching and the impact on the clinical interaction. Alternating use of two languages at the word phase, clause or sentences level with a clear break at phenomic system (word sounding) is defined as code switching. According to this article, code switching is shown to be a complex, rule governed phenomenon requiring a high degree of competence in more than one language. The purpose of this research is to determine ways to treat bilingual patients with Broca or Wernicke's aphasia.

The patient in the Reyes study is a second generation, is a 51-year-old Mexican-American right-handed man from El Paso, Texas. His parents spoke primarily Spanish and he learned to speak English and Spanish as a child. He completed the seventh grade, and married at age 18. He has six children between the ages 20 to 31. Mr. and Mrs. G spoke primarily in English to their children, but primarily Spanish with his wife, parents and siblings. He watches Spanish and English television programs and was employed as a construction worker. Mr. G was admitted to the hospital due to coronary artery disease. After bypass surgery, Mr. G suffered an embolic stroke, which is an obstruction of a blood vessel resulting in right hemiparesis, a weakness to the right side of the body, and expressive aphasia, difficulty transferring thoughts into words.

Mr. G's language skills were tested using a performance **Bilingual Aphasia Test (BAT)** to determine if his language skills were better in one language or the other, and to what extent. The test examines listening, speaking, reading and writing ability, and showed Mr. G performed similarly in Spanish and English. Where differences existed, performance was better in Spanish. Mr. G, therefore showed a synergistic pattern of language recovery, where both languages were equally impaired and progress in one language accompanied progress in the other language. Overall, Mr. G's performance was consistent with moderate to severe Broca's aphasia in both languages. Broca's aphasia is also called motor, expressive or anterior aphasia. Wernicki's aphasia is called sensory or posterior aphasia.

According to Reyes, it is important to recognize that the degree of bilingualism changes across time, topic and conflict. Further, the speech-pathologist must have a clear understanding of premorbid bilingualism before implementing treatment. For instance, the language used to treat often is the language spoken at home, the community setting and other factors need to be considered, such as, 1) premorbid language history; 2) educational and employment history; 3) family's choice of language, and 4) socio cultural language needs at discharge. For Mr. G, both languages were targeted. Mr. G would speak Spanish and say words in English and vice versa. The article also points out that not all bilingual speakers are proficient in each of their language and skilled at code switching. Knowing the patient's premorbid communication style and ability to code switch may be quite appropriate to use in the rehabilitative process for bilingual patients with aphasia.

While there are many factors to consider in the clinical management of the patient, this study used only one BAT to assess the patient's language impairment and did not talk about treatment modalities once the patient was assessed. There are at least 32 BAT subtests to assess reading, writing and translating skills. However, due to time constraints for this study only one BAT test was administered, the Bilingual Aphasia Test (Paradisi 1987). I believe the need for other testing was needed. Because Mr. G could code switch, he experienced other difficulties that impaired his ability to communicate. For instance, he articulated with frequent omissions of grammatical markers, such as noun and verb phrases were separated by distinct pauses. Sentence construction was severely compromised, as was his ability to repeat single words. Basically, Mr. G's verbal expression skills were impaired, where his auditory comprehension skills were better preserved. For example, he could point to objects with 100 percent accuracy and could follow most one to two-step commands.

Utilizing more than one BAT testing seems to be appropriate to better assess a patient's therapeutic needs and plan appropriate treatment. This study relates to the limited studies done among Hispanic bilingual people with aphasia.

Bilingual Aphasia and Subcortical-Cortical Lesions by Antonello, Bava, Cazzato, Moretti, Zivadinov, Zorzon, (2001).

The next review continues to examine effective ways to treat bilingual individuals affected by aphasia. According to the abstract on "Bilingual Aphasia Subcortical-Cortical lesions," psychologists treat bilingual Hispanics with the implicit memory procedure, which controls the subcortical structure. The subcortical is the portion of the brain immediately below the cerebral cortex of the brain. The cerebral cortex is the extensive outer layer of gray matter of the cerebral hemispheres largely responsible for higher brain functions, including sensation, vocabulary, muscle movement, thought, reason and memory. (Online available: www.dictionary.com). From this structure they are able to relate to the cortical structure, which depends on the cerebral cortex. By following this procedure pathologists treat the second language, which is dependent on the integrity of the explicit memory system, largely subserved by the cortical area. This area of subcortical - cortical area of studies and treatment relates to Broca'a Aphasia (also called motor, expressive, or anterior aphasia). This involves the anterior syndrome one area of Broca's study. This is damage in the left basal of the brain. The patterns of rehabilitation in Broca's aphasia and Wernicke's aphasia are related. Broca's aphasia, the subcortical study also relates to the second syndrome, which is Posterior Syndrome. The posterior syndrome is a lot like Wernicke's Aphasia except for the presence of hemiplegia. These two patterns relate to the central nervous system.

The topic of evaluation is about the subcortical - cortical lesions of the brain. A subcortical - cortical lesion is a condition due to a tumor in the front of the head, which caused damage to the cerebral cortex, which is like a bruise in the gray matter of the brain, and a tail like tissue; an appendage, obstructed the inflow of blood.

The abstract relates to the topic evaluation of aphasia in regards to variables that allow identifying, defining, and understanding how the subcortical - cortical affect the memory system and relates to the treatment for therapy through the implicit and explicit procedure which is administered to bilingual people with aphasia. Therefore, studying the subcortical - cortical lesions allows bilinguals to be considered as neurolinguistic models, which contribute to the understanding how the subcortical - cortical lesions of the language system relate while maintaining independent function.

The abstract points out how bilingual people with aphasia are given treatment, and what procedures are implemented and what patterns of rehabilitation are used to control memory. To know whether a patient is doing well is determined by measuring the patient's outcome. By using the implicit memory procedure, the patient was able to regain the use of his mother tongue as demonstrated at follow up visits.

The goal of treatment is for patients to regain the capacity to speak. The purpose of evaluating programs is to see how many programs are treating bilingual Hispanic patients with aphasia. The abstract illustrates limited studies were done among Hispanic bilingual people with aphasia.

In determining how to reach effective outcomes, I believe

psychologists first have to continue with follow up visits, and monitor the patient's progress by assessing the level of language performance, and explore other means of testing which have not been utilized.

Literature Reviews on Wernicke's Aphasia

In 1874, Carl Wernicke, a German neurologist, wrote about one of his patients who suffered from a comprehension disorder and was found to have a lesion in the posterior left temporal lobe of the brain. This area of the brain is responsible for perception, recognition and integration of sensory information. The affected part of the brain is now called Wernicke's area and the syndrome named Wernicke's aphasia. This syndrome is an acquired aphasia also known as sensory, receptive and jargon aphasia (**Davis 2000**).

Wernicke is considered a fluent aphasia, one of the aphasias that are caused by lesions inflicted by strokes or brain damage incurred through accidents to this area of the brain. Patients with Wernicke's aphasia have limited language comprehension, although they can produce language fluently (Davis 2000).

Wernicke's aphasia is considered the most unrelenting of the fluent aphasias Characteristics of Wernicke's aphasia are neologisms or made-up words, and confused, unintelligible language labeled "jargonaphasia" (Davis 2000).

Lesions in the left posterior frontal lobe around the area where motor functions take place cause another form of acquired aphasia, discovered by the physician Paul Broca in mid-nineteenth century. It is now called Broca's area and the aphasia is called Broca's aphasia. In short, Wernicke's area receives stimuli, whereas Broca's area emits responses (Davis 2000).

Surveys done on both Wernicke's and Broca's aphasics

show that Wernicke's patients are older than Broca's patients at the age of onset.

Wernicke's syndrome patients were, on average, in their 60's, while Broca's aphasics were in their 50's.

However, one researcher thought that this survey might be flawed by selection bias. It was assumed that Wernicke's patients suffered less damage and were able to survive longer than patients with Broca's aphasia who had extensive brain damage (Coppens 1991).

Strokes, tumors and accidents are the leading causes of acquired aphasia, although not every stroke, tumor or accident patient is subject to this condition. Patients with aphasia differ in their abilities to speak, to write, to read and to listen. Speech and writing are both affected by word finding difficulties. Reading comprehension is also often affected which in turn affects ability to listening. Consequently, aphasics may have very different levels of deficits in the ability to communicate (Davis 2000, p. 114).

Research indicates that with aphasia, in general, speech and writing are usually more impaired than is comprehension. Reading and writing abilities are generally more impaired than listening and speaking, depending upon whether the degree of aphasia is moderate or severe (Davis 2000).

Broca's is the most studied syndrome. Grodzinsky refers to it as "***the flagship of the neuropsychology of language***" (Grodinzsky 1991). One of the characteristics of Broca's aphasics is the inability to form normal, connected sentences known as agrammatism (Blunstein et al, 1998). It is associated with syntactic and semantic problems.

Despite extensive research into these deficits, there are disagreements about the findings. Researchers ascribed agrammatism to a separation of syntax, which is sentence structure, from other linguistic constituents of language.

These include: morphology the internal structure and form of words; semantics, which is the nature, structure and changes of the meaning of speech form (**Caramazza and Berndt 1978**). It was known as the "no-syntax hypothesis" (**Kolk and Van Grunsven 1985**). Other researchers disagree because it was not clear whether it pertains to syntactic knowledge or syntactic processes (Davis 2000).

Davis writes: "***Broca's aphasia is a swaggering flagship in a contentious sea***."

Some sensory disorders may stand-alone or may accompany aphasia, such as agnosia, the impairment of the ability to recognize a stimulus, even though sensory transmission is intact and dysarthria, the impairment of the ability to move the muscles used for speaking. This situation adds to the difficulties for the clinical diagnosis of aphasia. For example, a patient may have visual, auditory of tactile disorders, but that does not mean that the patient has aphasia nor does that rule out aphasia (Davis 2000). The physician makes a tentative diagnosis and refers the patient to a speech pathologist who determines if the patient is suffering from acquired aphasia or another kind of communication disorder (Davis 2000).

Speech pathologists first evaluate the oral-motor functions and communicative capacities to determine the diagnosis. Speech therapy is very difficult with Wernicke's patients because patients lack awareness of their speech deficits and overproduce "nonsense" speech (Davis 2000).

Treatment of Wernicke's aphasia is directed toward improving comprehension. Techniques must be used to keep the patient from talking excessively while in therapy. Patients must be trained to respond to the clinician's cues to remain quiet until the desired response is elicited by a "target" (Holland 1998), a picture of objects, numbers or other visual cues. Once this goal is met, the clinician begins introducing simple words and sentences that elicit comprehension.

Modeling techniques by clinicians have proved unsuccessful in stimulating and producing speech. Forcing speech interferes with auditory processes (Davis 2000). Patients lack awareness of their conditions and even an understanding of why they are in the clinic (**Sparks 1978**).

As opposed to Wernicke's patients who have overprotective speech, Broca's patients produce little speech. The "go strategy," a therapy to encourage patients with non-fluent aphasias to speak, is used with Broca's patients while the "stop strategy," a therapy to limit speech is used in therapy with fluent aphasics. To date, limited success and few treatment strategies have proven effective with fluent aphasias (**Holland 1978**).

Wernicke's aphasia, although one of the most difficult syndromes to treat, does not differ from other aphasias in the inability to master sentence structure (**Parisi and Pizzamiglio 1970**). In one study of the multiple meaning of words in sentences, four Wernicke subjects performed better than the test group with Broca's aphasia. The test used was the cross-modal semantic priming procedure (**Prather, et. al 1994**).

In a study of sentence formulation using pictures to elicit descriptions in words, Wernicke's subjects performed as well as neurologically intact subjects. However, Wernicke's participants produced more verbs than nouns and used indefinite words such as "this" and "here" than Broca's participants and participants who were neurologically intact (**Schwartz 1987**).

Most of the research in the field of aphasia has been done with Broca's aphasics. Davis (2000) reports: "Wernicke's aphasia has been swept up with Broca's in efforts to determine if aphasics include a broad double dissociation of semantic and syntactic functions" (Davis 2000).

Despite all the efforts of the scientific disciplines dealing with the brain since the turn of the last century - neurology, psychiatry, neuropsychiatry, to name a few - effective diagnostic and treatment modalities have yet to be discovered. In the 1920's speech disorders, including aphasia, were treated mainly with methods of speech correction used in public schools by speech pathologists. After World War II, veterans all over the world were treated by neurologists, psychologists and speech pathologists using therapies that were based on speech correction, classroom teaching and psychotherapy (Davis 2000).

By the end of the twentieth century veterans' life expectancies were increasing and the health problems related to aging brought aphasias to the forefront. Aphasias are now finally recognized as a unique communicative disorder (Davis 2000).

Aphasiology, the study of language disturbances caused by lesions in the brain, sprung out of neurology more than 100 years ago, but it was not until the 1970's that the processes of the mind were studied through a scientific approach (Davis 2000).

Aphasiologists differ in their views of the inner processes of communication. Some attribute encoding and decoding of the message to a function of neurons in the brain, while others believe encoding and decoding messages are the products of cognitive mental processes. These two different concepts of communication have brought two approaches to the scientific studies of communications. The aphasiologist studies the brain irrespective of the cognitive dysfunction. The neuropsychologist studies cognitive disorders, (Davis 2000) irrespective of the cognitive dysfunction. The neuropsychologist studies cognitive disorders, (Davis 2000).

Neurologists explain communication in terms of the brain. Location and magnitude of the damage in the brain accounts for aspects and degrees of malfunction of neurogenic communication. The implications of these finding pose questions of treatment, because the clinician must have knowledge of the nervous system and its pathology (Brookshire 1997).

Through scientific research, clinical aphasiology attempts to unfold the many questions surrounding aphasias for the purposes of description and explanation. Aside from its diagnostic function, clinical aphasiology attempts to create effective treatments that will help the aphasics and their families to cope with the difficulties of this disorder (Davis 2000).

Experimental psychologists refer to the mind as cognition, "the collection of mental processes and activities used in perceiving remembering, thinking and understanding (Ashcroft 1994). Cognitive science can contribute knowledge through the study of dysfunction. Neuroscience can contribute through brain investigations to the etiology of aphasia (Davis 2000).

For the last three decades new means including standardized tests have been created: Porch Index of Communicative Ability (Porch 1971); Boston Diagnostic Aphasia Examination (Goodglass 1972); Western Aphasia Battery (Kertesz 1982); and Neurosensory Center Comprehensive Examination for Aphasia (Spreen 1969). Daily Living (Holland 1980). The Token Test assesses certain characteristics of the aphasic's receptive disturbances (**Derenzi, Vignolo 1962**).

The diverse characteristics of the syndromes presuppose diverse impairments of the different psycholinguistic processes that in turn pose questions for therapy. Can a single plan of action be suitable for the treatment of aphasia? Will it be effective?

"Clinical professionals will be especially responsive if psycholinguistic paradigms identify impairments reliably and the diagnosis makes a difference in treatment accuracy and efficiency." (Davis 2000).

Conclusion

Patients with a learning disturbance, aphasia, may not outgrow their disability. However, they can learn to adapt by developing their personal strengths and work around their disability.

For many individuals, the process to recovery after an injury to the brain may take years or the person may never be fully complete. With the proper ongoing training and compassion, creating a supportive environment can help to develop the patient as a unique individual.

There are many factors that interfere with obtaining adequate care and treatment for Hispanic bilinguals with aphasia. From my interviews with patients, the following five points were expressed: 1) patients stated how expensive tests are and that most insurances do not cover costs. 2) There are very few therapists, and 3) family members cannot always take patients for needed services. 4) Transportation availability and costs are other factors, and 5) therapists do not do home visits.

From the readings, it is important for speech pathologists to measure the level of progress of the treatment. The patient should be tested at different intervals and then appropriate treatment applied that will also give the patient a sense of progress to validate prescribed treatment. By following this type of procedure, it should verify the reliability and effectiveness of the tools used and prescribed treatment.

In conclusion, the programs that offer rehabilitative care

should continuously monitor and evaluate the patient's progress to establish better means of patient care. Additionally, rehabilitative programs should explore government funding possibilities to assist people with aphasia and thereby provide continued care for those with limited or no insurance coverage.

CHAPTER III

SUBJECT, MATERIALS, AND PROCEDURES

This chapter will begin to investigate / explore the patterns of rehabilitation for Hispanic bilingual patients with aphasia. The study will focus on how neurologists and speech pathologists can help bilingual Hispanics with aphasia when the ability to understand language and to translate thoughts into words is impaired as a result of a traumatic brain injury, stroke or disease.

The goal of treatment is for patients to regain the capacity to speak. The purpose of evaluating programs is to see how many programs are treating bilingual Hispanic patients with aphasia. The abstract illustrates limited studies were done among Hispanic bilingual people with aphasia.

In determining how to reach effective outcomes, it's believed that psychologists first have to continue with follow up visits, and monitor the patient's progress by assessing the level of language performance, and explore other means of testing which have not been utilized.

Subjects Broca's Aphasia

Broca's aphasia is usually Broca's Aphasia seen following damage to the posterior inferior frontal lobe and causes paralysis of one side of the body (hemiplegia) or hemipareis, weakness of one side of the body. For right-handed individuals this would almost always affect the right side of the body because the lesions that cause aphasia are almost always left-hemishere lesions and motor control is contralateral, occurring on or acting in conjunction with similar parts on the opposite side of the brain.

Characteristics of Broca's Aphasia

Broca's aphasia is also called motor, expressive, or anterior aphasia. The characteristics of aphasia or symptoms affect speech that is non-fluent, labored and halting. The intonation and stress patterns are deficient, and misarticulations are prominent. Broca'a speech is often telegraphic, which are short abrupt words and agrammatical that are no function words like conjunctions, articles or prepositions. The auditory comprehension of a person with Broca's aphasia is usually much better than their speech. According to an article online by Gliesche, Sherny T. (No date). Aphasia. Archived file at
http:/I.imssf.org/aphasia/htm.

Wernicke's Aphasia

Wernicke's aphasia is produced by lesions in the posterior third of the superior temporal gyrus, Wernicke's area, in the distribution of the inferior division of the middle cerebral artery. Additionally, Wernicke's aphasia usually occurs in the auditory association area of the left hemisphere deficit involving the temporal-partial region of the brain. Also, known as Global aphasia because the patient has difficulty, both in understanding spoken words as well as in common autonomic tasks in response to visual cues rather than responding to specific spoken commands. (Gliesche, No date).

Wernicke is considered a fluent aphasia, one of the aphasias that are caused by lesions inflicted by strokes or brain damage incurred through accidents to this area of the brain. Patients with Wernicke's aphasia have limited language comprehension, although they can produce language fluently Wernicke's aphasia is considered the most unrelenting of the fluent aphasias. (Davis 2001).

Characteristics of Wernicke's Aphasia

Wernicke's aphasia is also called the sensory, receptive, or posterior aphasia. Characteristics of Wernicke's aphasia are neologisms or made-up words, and confused, unintelligible language labeled "jargonaphasia" (Davis 2001). The person with Wernicke's aphasia often is notable handicapped by an inability to process single words through the auditory modality. This is why picture to word matching skills help to correctly read picture single words aloud. Other characteristics include fluent speech, except for pauses that may occur as the patient experiences word-find difficulty. The rate, intonation, and stress are normal, but speech sounds are empty and lacking in content and meaning. Patients substitute one word for another, such as "table" for "chair," is common in the speech of those with Wernicke's aphasia. Auditory comprehension for example, understanding what is said to them, is usually quite poor, according to (**Gliesche** No Date).

Classification of Aphasia

A procedure used to classify aphasia is the aphasia classification system used most commonly by aphasiologists include the following syndromes, broadly grouped as "cortical" or "subcortical" according to the major site of the responsible brain lesion:

"Cortical" Syndromes

Broca°s aphasia Wernicke's aphasia Conduction aphasia Anomic aphasia Transcortical motor aphasia Transcortical sensory aphasia Global aphasia

"Subcortical" Syndromes

Anterior capsular/putaminal aphasia Posterior capsular/putaminal aphasia Global capsular/putaminal aphasia Thalamic aphasia

As many as 80% of patients whose aphasia results from a stroke can be classified according to this system. Some unclassifiable forms of aphasia may be accounted for by such factors as unusual combinations of lesion sites within the left hemisphere, atypical cerebral dominance with left-handedness or ambidexterity, or a positive neurological history, which might include previous strokes, carotid (chief artery or pair of arteries that pass up the neck and supply the head) insufficiency, or substance abuse. Because these same factors may influence recovery patterns, this information should be obtained for all patients, even those whose aphasia is easily classifiable." (**Heim-Estabrooks 1983**, p.23).

The aphasia classification system described relates primarily to the acquired language disorders resulting from left cerebral stroke. In most cases there will be a history of sudden onset, often associated with right-sided weakness or paralysis, following which these symptoms become stable or improve. If instead there is slow onset of speech/language problems with continued deterioration, then an etiology other than stroke (e.g., dementia, brain tumor, vasculitis, encephalitis) should be considered and investigated. (**Helm-Estabrooks 1983**, p.23).

Bilingual Aphasia

Bilingual Aphasia refers to the Subcortical-Cortical lesions. Psychologists treat bilingual Hispanics with the implicit memory procedure, which controls the subcortical structure. The subcortical is the portion of the brain immediately below the cerebral cortex of the brain. The cerebral cortex is the extensive outer layer of gray matter of the cerebral hemispheres largely responsible for higher brain functions, including sensation, vocabulary, muscle movement, thought, reason and memory. (Online available: http://www.dictionary.com). From this structure they are able to relate to the cortical structure, which depends on the cerebral cortex. By following this procedure pathologists treat the second language, which is dependent on the integrity of the explicit memory system, largely subserved by the cortical area. This area of subcortical - cortical area of studies and treatment relates to Broca's Aphasia (also called motor, expressive, or anterior aphasia). This involves the anterior syndrome one area of Broca's study. This is damage in the left basal of the brain. The patterns of rehabilitation in Broca's aphasia and Wernicke's aphasia are related. Broca's aphasia, the subcortical study also relates to the second syndrome, which is Posterior Syndrome. The posterior syndrome is a lot like Wernicke's Aphasia except for the presence of hemiplegia. These two patterns relate to the central nervous system.

The topic of evaluation is about the subcortical - cortical lesions of the brain. A subcortical - cortical lesion is a condition due to a tumor in the front of the head, which caused damage to the cerebral cortex, which is like a bruise in the gray matter of the brain, and a tail like tissue; an appendage, obstructed the inflow of blood.

Neuroanatomy

An introduction to the study and treatment of aphasia must first consider the neural basis of language, that is, the normal apparatus. However, a comprehensive map of brain language relationships is far from fully developed, and new techniques of brain imaging have considerably modified classical teachings. Nevertheless, much of what had been taught in the past retains current clinical validity, such as that lesions in the "zone of language" in the left hemisphere of most right-handed people usually will produce aphasia. However, many additional regions of the brain are known to contribute to language function, including right hemispheric and subcortical structures. (**Helm-Estabrooks 1983**, p.23).

To understand the anatomy of language, one should have a general understanding of neuroanatomy. From the effected organ (e.g., muscle) inward, the following components of the nervous system should be considered: peripheral nerves, spinal cord, brain stem, cerebellum, subcortical nuclear structures (subcortical gray matter), subcortical white matter (association pathways, commissures, corpus callosum), and cortex. At the same time, one must have a picture of how these various anatomical systems are organized regionally (e.g., limbic system, frontal lobe, temporal lobe, etc.).

Specific neuroanatomical structures never function in complete isolation from other parts of the brain. All complex cognitive skills, such as language, arise from the interaction of multiple anatomical regions, that is, overlapping and interconnected neural networks widely distributed throughout the brain, carrying out their specific neural functions both sequentially and in parallel. The concept of parallel distributed processing (POP), popular in contemporary science, provides a useful metaphor for the understanding of higher cortical functions in humans. The simplest language task depends on a complex interaction of the reticular activating system, subcortical nuclear structures, right hemisphere, subcortical white matter, and left-hemispheric "zone of language."

Neuroanatomical Structures

A. Basic Components

Nerve cells (neurons) comprise the basic elements, the building blocks, of the nervous system. Each neuron consists of a cell body and branching processes called nerve fibers. Dendrites are short nerve fibers that receive electrochemical impulses and transport these impulses toward the cell body. An axon is a long nerve fiber that generally transports impulses away from the cell body (see Fig. 3).

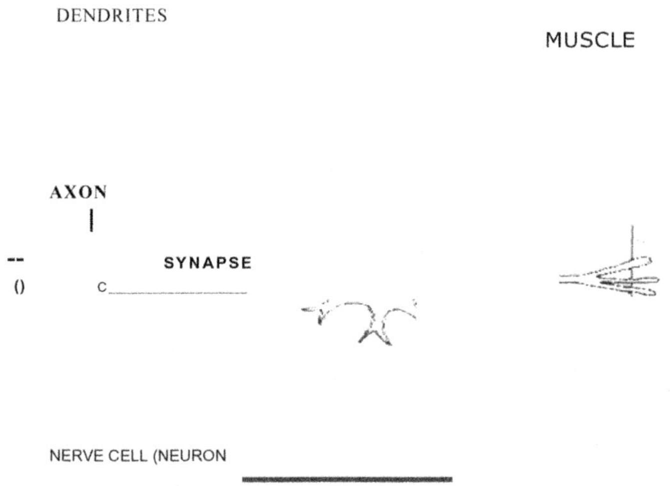

FIG. 3. Neurons

NERVE CELL (NEURON)

Neural transmission refers to the transfer of electrochemical impulses (or "information") from one neuron to another. Neurotransmitters are chemical substances, such as dopamine or acetylcholine, that may be transferred from one neuron to another, or that may facilitate or interfere with neural transmission. Neural transmission takes place at a synapse or junction between two neurons. Often the axon of one neuron connects with the dendrites of another neuron. In such a transmission pathway, the afferent fiber is the one carrying a neural impulse toward the cell body, while the efferent fiber is the one carrying the impulse away from a cell body.

Neurons (cell body and fibers) generally are organized in clusters. A cluster of nerve cell bodies located within the brain or spinal cord is called a nucleus. A cluster of nerve cell bodies located outside the brain and spinal cord is called a ganglon. A cluster of nerve fibers within the brain or spinal cord that has a common origin and common final end point may be called a tract, column, commissure, fasciculus, or pathway. Gray matter refers to regions of the brain or spinal cord containing clusters of nerve cell bodies. In a postmortem examination of the brain, clusters of nerve cell bodies appear gray, in contrast with collections of white or cream-colored nerve fibers, which are called white matter. The cerebral cortex consists of layers of nerve cells, appears gray in color, and is included with cerebra nuclei as the gray matter of the brain. (See Figure 4).

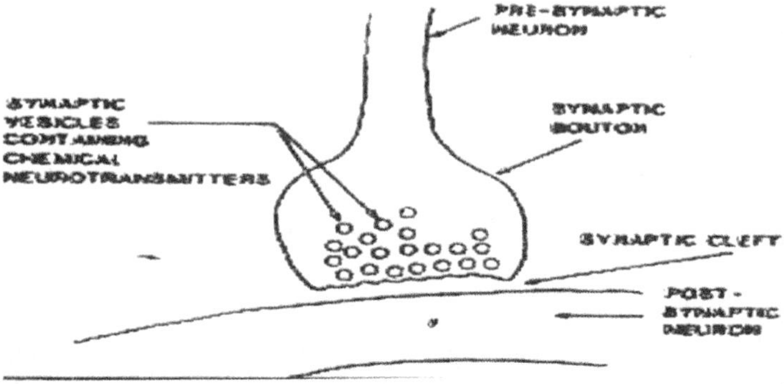

Fig. 4. Chemical synaptic neurotransmission. Chemical neurotransmitters are released from synaptic vesicles in the presynaptic neuron, pass across the synaptic cleft, and excite or inhibit the postsynaptic neuron.

Figure 4. Chemical synaptic neurotransmission. Chemical neurotransmitters are released from synaptic vesicles in the presynaptic neuron, pass across the synaptic cleft, and excite or inhibit the postsynaptic neuron.

B. Central Nervous System

The central nervous system includes the brain (gray and white matter of the cerebral hemispheres, brain stem, and cerebellum) and spinal cord. The brain, about the size of a small grapefruit, weighs about 1.250 grams and is composed of an estimated 15 billion neurons plus supporting cells.

C. Spinal Cord

The spinal cord travels through the vertebral column carrying neural impulses from the periphery to the brain for further analysis and from the brain to the periphery to produce responses. Spinal nerves appear in pairs, one on each side of the cord. There are 31 of these pairs: 8 cervical, 12 thoracic, 5 lumbar, 5 sacral, and 1 coccygeal.

D. Brain Stem

The brain stem is divided into three segments: medulla, pons, and midbrain. The medulla oblongata, or medulla, is the continuation of the spinal cord through the base of the skull. This portion of the brain stem contains nuclei for the cranial nerves responsible for movements of the tongue, orpharynx, larynx, and diaphragm. Cough and gag reflexes also are mediated at this level of the brain.

The pons is continuous with the medulla, and the midbrain is continuous with the pons. These segments of the brain contain cranial nerve nuclei for eye movements, facial expression, facial sensation, and hearing.

E. Cerebellum

The cerebellum sits like a roof over the brain stem and is composed of a surface layer of gray matter and an inner core of white matter and cerebellar nuclei. The cerebellum consists of two large lateral masses, the cerebellar hemispheres (to be distinguished from the cerebral hemispheres) and a narrow midline portion, the vermis. The cerebellum is responsible for integrating or coordinating muscle groups throughout the body. To function normally, motor activity must flow with a smooth, regular, well-timed, well-coordinated rhythm. The cerebellum maintains this rhythm. Abnormalities of cerebellar function may affect the muscles of the glossopharyngeal apparatus, producing speech disorders such as dysarthria or ataxia.

F. Subcortical Gray Matter

Deep within the cerebral hemispheres are several collections (nerve cell bodies that comprise the subcortical gray matter serving a variety of sensory, motor, and integrative functions. These structures include the diencephalon and the basal ganglia. The diencephalon consists primarily of the thalamus and hypothalamus and their connections. The basal ganglia consist primarily of the caudate nucleus, putamer globus pallidus, and amygdala.

Lesions of basal ganglia have been linked to symptoms found within aphasic syndromes. Small bilateral lesions of the basal ganglia are often the cause of hypophonic speech. Dysarthria may result from damage to basal ganglia; if the damage is unilateral, the dysarthria is usually transient. Nonfluent and fluent aphasias as well as global aphasia can result from left-hemispheric lesions in the region of the basal ganglia. It has not been ascertained whether these subcortical aphasic syndromes result from damage to subcortical nuclei (gray matter), pathways (white matter), or both.

Cortico-cortical association fibers connect different regions of the cortex to each other. In his 1965 paper "Disconnexion syndromes in Animals and Man," Norman Geschwind provided a speculative explanation of the process of naming based in large part on the availability in the human brain of cortico-cortical association fibers. Of particular interest for the anatomy of language are the superior longitudinal fasciculus, a white matter pathway connecting posterior cortical sensory bundle of nerve fibers arching from the auditory association area in the temporal lobe (Wernicke's area) and joining the superior longitudinal fasciculus, eventually making its way to the frontal motor association cortex for the muscles of the glossopharyngeal apparatus (Broca's area). Several lesions in the brain can produce the aphasic feature of impaired repetition of speech; one of these lesions is in the arcuate fasciculus.

New brain imaging techniques have revealed the importance of subcortical structures in language. It seems that cortico sub-cortical white matter pathways may be equally important. Because white matter pathways into neural networks that subserve language function connect cortical gray matter and subcortical nuclei, lesions in these white matter pathways may lead to aphasic phenomena.

Instrumentation

Brain injury appears to affect from 132 to 367 people per 100,000. Traditional methods for diagnosing mild head injury are taking the medical history, neurologic exam; perform CAT scan and MRI, magnetic radiology imaging, standard EEG and neuropsychological testing. These tests often show normal test results even through patients complain of significant neurocognitive dysfunctions.

The Glasgow Coma Scare of 13 is used as criteria for loss of consciousness and amnesia to know the length of the of Unconsciousness. Although this particular test is used for both head injuries and stroke victims, many clinicians find this test to be of little value. (**Hoffman, Hicks, Schwaniger, Stockdale, (2001)**).

In the **Reyes Study** of a bilingual Hispanic who suffered a stroke, the **Bilingual Aphasia Test** assessed the patient's language impairment. There are an additional 32 BAT subtests to use to assess reading, writing and translating skills for bilingual Hispanic patients with aphasia.

Psychologists treat bilingual Hispanics with the implicit memory procedure by first diagnosing the patient with a Battery of Repetition Tests. By following this procedure pathologist treat the second language (English), which is dependent on the integrity of the explicit memory system.

All aphasics have problems naming objects. The first step as with a bilingual Hispanic patient is to establish the presence of a naming disorder called anomia. The process is as follows: The patient has a stroke, and a Battery of Naming Tests is done. Some patients may have a low frequency scale, such as naming a telescope, and some may have a high frequency scale, naming body parts and colors. Abnormal naming performance assist with identifying an aphasic patient.

Determining speech fluency is subdivided into two forms, fluent aphasia and nonfluent aphasia, which is based on characteristics of conversational speech. Fluent aphasia can be exhibited by fluent easily pronounced speech; lack of meaningful words, i.e. nonspecific, vague or irrelevant; excessive talking words that are jumbled together, like an alphabet salad, or putting words together that do not make sense, sound or word substitution, decreased ability to name pictures and objects, and also have difficulty writing. A person exhibiting nonfluent aphasia has difficulty producing speech or writing. A person exhibiting nonfluent aphasia has difficulty producing speech or repeating words; elimination of non-meaningful words due to the effort of speaking; decreased ability to name pictures and objects; searching for sounds with various mouth movements, and difficulty writing.

The Boston Assessment of Severe Aphasia can also test patients. For example, "Close your eyes," "how are you today?" The responses are recorded which is later judged objectively from a transcription. The session should be tape recorded for careful analysis. This test delineates the nature of auditory comprehension deficit. Afterwards the clinician needs to decide whether the existing deficit interferes with the patient's daily life, and if it does, then social skills and adapting to environment will be diagnosed and evaluated.

A variety of battery tests were conducted, such as, Rating a Conversational Speech Sample, which determines conversational measures that fall either at the center (a rating of 4) or to the left of center, the diagnosis is nonfluent aphasia. The factors are phrase length beginning with a single word up to 7 or more words, substantive/functor word balance; grammatical form ranging from none to normal range; paraphasias rate to frequent; speech prosody - severely impaired to normal, and articularory agility - severely impaired to normal. If most of the ratings are to the right of center, a diagnosis of fluent aphasia is made. In some syndromes, however, one of these parameters may deviate from the fluent/nonfluent feature dichotomy. See figure 5.

NonfluentAphasia	Y	Fluent Aphasia	
Poor Auditorv Comerehension	Good Auditorv Comprehension	Poor Auditorv Comprehension	Good Auditorv Comprehension
Global	Broca's	Wernicke's	Coniuction
	Transcortical Motor	Transcortical Sensorv	Anomic

Battery of Auditory Comprehension Tests identifies single word objects (high to low frequency) and actions (high to low frequency), includes letters, numbers, colors and body parts. Following commands: single-step, naturalistic actions, two-three-four-step, and unusual actions. Understanding questions related to personal information, impersonal information, everyday stories, and paragraphs of obscure facts:

The treatment provided based on the various diagnostic and battery tests showed very little progress in all treatments. The patient after a number of days returned to the first stage of treatment in ability to change thoughts into words. Because of the damage to the front lobal area of the brain, one can only speak to the person with aphasia very slowly, one word at a time following the one step command.

In the process of recuperation the physical state of the particular patient plays a significant role, which involves the nature of the lesion and the cortical function. At times the patient seems to be ready, but at other times unready to produce integrations necessary for use in language. In short, aphasia therapy helps facilitate new pathways for successful integration of language, in other words the individual is ready to be productive at that time through stimulation. Facilitation is defined in this respect as the ability to increase the flow of energy into the system which permits it to form new integrations for language, utilizing the nervous tissue present which seems incapable of spontaneous function. (Wepman 1972).

Treatment therapy is a long process that must be continued at home with family members and with a speech pathologist. The ways to communicate with a patient with aphasia is to wait for the person to finish speaking. Do not finish the sentence for them. Be sensitive to noise and keep voice in a normal to low tone. Be open to different ways of communicating, such as gestures, writing and facial expressions. Always verify that you are communicating successfully with the patients, with a simple, "yes," "no" response.

Progress takes time and insurance companies need to become aware of aphasia as a language disorder that takes patients along time to show improvement.

Procedures

Treatment possibilities would include alternate ways to communicate and treatment to improve the areas of difficulty. To facilitate treatment the therapist begins by understanding when the patient is ready for treatment and motivates the patient into treatment.

A speech language pathologist helps the patient with specialized treatment for speech, language and swallowing disorder (dysphagia). Speech language pathologists may use computer technology, ultrasound procedures, voice or language exercises or other training. For many, the treatments can restore communication skills. Certified speech pathologists receive a Master's degree from an accredited program, conduct a clinical fellowship year and pass a national examination to receive their Certificate of Clinical Competence in speech-language pathology from the American Speech-Language-Heading Association (ASHA). This information provided by the American Speech Language Hearing Association.

Treatment for stroke and for mild closed head injuries has included early intervention, education, family and professional support, group therapy, individual psychotherapy, marital and family therapy, stress reduction therapy, coping skills training, multidisciplinary pain management, neuropsychological rehabilitation, vocational counseling, work skills training and multidisciplinary psychological rehabilitation (Howard, 1993).

CHAPTER IV

RESULTS, DISCUSSION, AND CONCLUSIONS

Findings

Aphasia cannot be cured, because there are no medicines or drugs known to cure aphasia, as yet. Surgery is successful in those occasions where pressure from a brain tumor or a hematoma impacts a critical speech center. Surgery is not useful in cases of aphasia following stroke, which represent the vast majority of instances. Speech therapy is often provided to persons with aphasia, but does not guarantee a "cure." The purpose of speech therapy is to help the patient to fully utilize remaining skills and to learn compensatory means of communication.

Qualitative/Results

The case of Martin Exeter, a university professor and lecturer who suffered from Wernicke's aphasia after a stroke, was able to live a relatively normal life with treatment. He was able to travel and lecture again. During his treatment, he received a great deal of support from his wife, colleagues, and friends. He could have improved even more, had it not been for a brain tumor that developed later and ended his life. (Davis 2000).

Discussion

The patient, the therapist, and the therapeutics have three sources that must be considered in formulating a working model for the recovery of aphasia.

Of primary importance is the patient himself, his/her personality and intellectual propensities. Some researchers differ in opinions regarding the personality structure or the intellectual potentiality as factors that have any effects in aphasia recovery. Various opinions claim that brain damage causes change in personality making aphasics very much alike. Others claim that only overt behavior changes, while the basic personality remains the same. The same applies for intellectual ability following cortical damage. It is claimed by some researches that the ability to abstract deteriorates; however, scientific evidence is yet to be obtained to support this claim.

This research on aphasia allowed ways to investigate /explore the patterns of rehabilitation of aphasia. The goal is to understand how therapists could help bilingual Hispanic with aphasia. Aphasia has no cultural boundaries. Any human being can be stricken with aphasia whether it is man, woman or child. Aphasia is a condition caused by a stroke, and once a person's brain is damaged there lives are no longer the same.

The purpose of the study was to find out what type of treatment is given to bilingual Hispanics. It's not that psychologist, or speech pathologists have not been successful treating bilingual Hispanics, the problem has been treating the bilingual Hispanic patient who has a language disorder.

In the Reyes case study (1997), bilingual Hispanic patients with aphasia focused on bilingualism and code switching. In Reyes' study, code switching is shown to be a complex, rule governed phenomenon requiring a high degree of competence in more than one language. The purpose of this research is to determine ways to treat bilingual Hispanic patients with Broca and Wernicke's aphasia. It is important to recognize beneficial treatment for bilingual Hispanic patients. Speech pathologists need to understand the precondition of the patient before implementing treatment. For instance, which language is used for treatment, English or Spanish?

Limitations and Implementations

There are limited studies among bilingual Hispanic people with aphasia. The purpose of the study was to determine what type of aphasia affected bilingual Hispanics, and what kind of rehabilitation was provided. Due to the confidentiality law, the ethnographic study could not be performed. The study was continued by using existing data, which was provided by a therapist at an urban facility.

Patients with a learning disturbance, aphasia, may not outgrow their disability. However, they can learn to adapt by developing their personal strengths and work around their disability. For many individuals, the process to recovery after an injury to the brain may take years or the person may never be fully complete. With the proper ongoing training and compassion, creating a supportive environment can help to develop the patient as a unique individual.

Summary

Investigating / exploring the patterns of rehabilitation of aphasia for Bilingual Hispanics, showed improved language performance by repeating words, sounds, viewing videos, and picture cards in addition to utilizing the Battery of Repetition Tests as an ongoing assessment tool. Further, it is important to understand the anatomical functions of the brain in order to work with a patient with communication disorder caused by a stroke, brain injury or disease.

It is interesting to learn that by using a battery test called implicit memory procedure; the battery test has benefited Hispanic bilingual patients. In recognizing the area of the brain affected, the implicit memory procedure can be used as a modality of treatment for bilingual Hispanic patients. It is fair to state that this test is a positive approach to treating bilingual Hispanic patients with language disorders. By identifying and isolating the damaged area and knowing how it interacts with other parts of the brain structure, therapists can then become better at diagnosing and treating bilingual aphasic patients. Damaged areas of the brain can effect sensation, vocabulary, muscle movement, thought, reason and memory. The Reyes study pointed out that the implicit memory procedure is one of many repetitions of battery test that can be used to work with bilingual Hispanic patients with aphasia. Alternative approaches can work with bilingual Hispanic aphasia patients. The key to maintaining the level of therapy in order to rehabilate a patient with aphasia, is repeating and practicing specific exercises of treatment daily and encouraging the patient to continue treatment at home.

In summary, stimulation, the actions of the individuals around the aphasics that awakens the patients ' interest to react, facilitation, the strengthening of the drives that motivate the actions, and motivation, the patients bundle of goal-directed behavior constitute the fortress that empowers aphasia patients to become independent. Unless the patients regain the wholesome self-concept once lost and become functional members in society again aphasia therapy cannot be claimed to work effectively. The only way for success is to put to work the concepts of stimulation, facilitation, and motivation. Programs that offer rehabilitative care should continuously monitor and evaluate the patient's progress to establish better means of patient care. Rehabilitative programs should explore government funding possibilities to assist people with aphasia and thereby provide continued care for those with limited or no insurance coverage.

Therapists need to look at the patient's premorbid history, educational and employment history, family's choice of language and socio cultural language needed at discharge. Bilingual Hispanics speakers are proficient in English and Spanish because they have the ability to code switch from Spanish to English, and vice versa. Therapists need to look at which language the patient is able to begin his/her therapy.

The therapist plays a crucial role in the recovery of aphasia. His/her role in the treatment process requires profound knowledge of how the cortex works as well as a keen sense to detect the patient's readiness for stimulation to respond to the treatment. He/she should be able to recognize to what degree the patient can receive stimulation, in what area of language he can be stimulated, and what kind of response is generated by different kinds of stimulation. The therapist must be concerned with the patient's personality, needs and desires which are more important than the different therapies that may or may not prove effective in stimulating and educating aphasics. The treatment should be geared to stimulate the recovery of the ability to integrate the language lost and the ability to learn new vocabulary.

References

Alavi A., Ding, X.S., D'Esposito, M., Grossman, M., Hughes E., Mickanin,

J., Onishi, K, Reivich, M. (1996). Progressive nonfluent aphasia: language, cognitive, and P. F. measures contrasted with probable Alzheimer's disease. Journal of Cognitive Neuroscience. V8 n2 p135(20). Massachusetts Institute of Technology.

Anderson, P.L., Meier-Hedde, R. (2001). Early Case Reports of Dyslexia in the United States and Europe. Journal of Learning Disabilities. V34 it pg. Thomson Corporation Company.

Antonello, R.M ., Bava, A Cazzato G.Moretti, R., Zivadinov, R Zorzon, M. Torre, P. (2001). Bilingual Aphasia and Subcortical-Cortical Lesions. Perceptual and Motor Skills. V92 i3 p803. Thomson Corporation Company.

Aphasia. The Gale Encyclopedia of Childhood and Adolescence.

Aphasia. (2001). National Aphasia Association. Fact Sheet. p I. New York. Available: http://www.aphasia.org.

Barrett. K. (2001). Aphasia. Gale Encyclopedia of Medicine. [Online] Available: http://www.findarticles.com/cf 1/g2 00517/p1/article.jhtml?term=aphasia.

Bates, Devescovi, A., Wulfeck, B., (2001). Psycholinguistics: A Cross-Language Perspective. Annual Review of Psychology. p369. Thomson Corporation Company.

Bliss M., (2001). Tip-of-the-tongue experiences. The Lancet. V357 19251 p236. Thomson Corporation Company.

Blumstein, S.E., Byma G, Kurowiki, K, Hourihan, J. Brown, T., and Hutchinson, A. (1985). Online processing of filler-gap constructions in aphasia. Brain and Language, 61, 149 - 168).

Brookshire, R.H. (1997). Introduction to neurogenic communication disorders (5thEd.) St. Louis, Mo. Mosby.

Caramaua, A., and Berndt, R.S. 1978. Semantic and syntactic processes in aphasia: a review of literature. Psychological Bulletin, 85, 898-918).

Coppens, P. (1991). Why are Wernicke's aphasia patients older than Broca's? A critical view of the hypothesis. Aphasiology, 5, 279 - 290

Davis, G.A. (2000). Aphasiology: disorders and clinical practice. Boston: Allyn and Bacon, 1, 2, 3, 4, 5, 9-10, 11-12, 16, 19, 36, 37, 39, 92, 98, 106-107, 114, 115, 118, 280.

Dictionary. (2002). (Online available: www.dictionary.com).

Donnan, G.A., Carey, L.M., Saling, M.M. (1999). More (or less) on Broca. The

Lancet. V353 19158 p 1031 (1). Thomson Corporation Company. Freeman, Y.S., Freeman, D.E. (1992). Language Learning Takes Place. Whole to Part. Whole Language for Second Language Learners. (p13).

Heineman Press. New Hampshire.

Gilbride, D., Stensrud, R., Ehlers, C., Evans, E., Peterson, C. (2000). Employers'

Attitudes toward hiring persons with disabilities and vocational rehabilitation services. Journal of Rehabilitation. Vol. 66, Issue 4. (p17?23). Alexandria, MD.

Goodglass, H. and Kaplan E. E. (1972). Boston Diagnostic Aphasia Examination. Philadelphia: Lea and Gebiger.

Grodzinsky, Y. (1991). There is an entity called agrammatic aphasia. Brain and Language, 41, 555 - 564

Helm-Estabrooks, N. (1983). Neuroanatomy of Language. Manual of Aphasia Therapy. Foundation of Aphasia Rehabilitation. (pp. 3-16). New York: Academic Press.

Hiebert, E. H. (1991). Diversity and Constancy in Human Thinking: Critical Literacy as Amplifier of an Intellect and Experience. Literacy for a Diverse Society. Perspectives, Practices, and Policies. (p 44). Teachers College Press. New York, NY.

Hillis, A. E., Caramazza, A. (1995). Cognitive and neural mechanisms underlying visual and semantic processing: implications from "optic aphasia." Journal of Cognitive Neuroscience. (1995). p 457(22). Massachusetts Institute of Technology.

Holland, A.L. (1998) why can't clinicians talk to aphasic adults? Comments on supported conversation for adults with aphasia: methods and resources for training conversational partners. Aphasiology. 12, 844 - 846.

Krashen, S., Terre!, T.D. Providing Input for Acquisition. The Natural Approach: Language Acquisition in the Classroom. 2nd Edition. (pp. 57-79). Alemany Press. New York, NY.

Kreutzer, J.S., Witol, A.D. (1996). Supported Employment as an Option for Return to Competitive Employment. Le Magazine. Vol. 4, No. 1. (p8, 10-11).

Kertesz, A. (1982) Western aphasia Battery, New York: Grune and Stratton. Kolk, H. and van Grunsven, M.M. (1985) Agramatism as a variable phenomenon. Cognitive Neuropsychology, 2, 347 - 384.

Meairs, S., Timpe, L., Beyer, J., Hennerici, M. (2000). Acute aphasia and hemiplegi during karate training. The

Lancet. V 356 19223 p40. Thomson Corporation Company.

Moretti, R., Bava, A., Torre, P., Antonello, R.M., Zorzon, M., Zivadinov, R., Cazzato, G. (2001). Bilingual Aphasia and Subcortical-Cortical Lesions. Perceptual and Motor Skills. V92 i3 p 803. Thomson Corporation Company.

McNellis, M.G., Blumstein, S.E. (2001). Self-Organizing Dynamics of Lexical Access in Normals and Aphasics. Journal of Cognitive Neuroscience. V13 i2 p151. Massachusetts Institute of Technology.

Reyes, B.A., Peterson, C.S. (1997). Hispanic Americans: Culture, communication, and clinical management. In G.L. Wallace (Ed.), Multicultural Neurogenics: A resource for speech-language pathologists providing services to neurologically impaired adults from culturally and linguistically diverse backgrounds. p165-191. San Antonio TX. Communication Skill Builders.

Senior K:(2001). Angiogenesis and functional recovery demonstrated after minor stroke. The Lancet. v3ORNO 58 i9284 p817. Thomson Corporation Company.

Sarno, M:(1972) Aphasia Select Reading. New York. University of Medicine. Meredith Corporation.

Tran, M. (2001). Memory loss. Gale Encyclopedia of Alternative Medicine. [Online] Available:

http://www.findarticles.com/cf 1 /g2 00517/p 1 /article. jhtml?term=aphasia. Webster, M. (1991) Webster Ninth New Collegiate Dictionary. Merriam-Webster Inc., Publishers Springfield, Massachusetts, U.S.A.

ABSTRACT

This research on aphasia was to investigate / explore the patterns of rehabilitation of aphasia. The goal was to understand how could therapists help bilingual Hispanics with aphasia. Aphasia has no cultural boundaries. Any human being can be stricken with aphasia whether it is man, woman or child. Aphasia is a condition caused by neurological damage or disease to the brain, which affects a person's ability to communicate as a result of a brain injury, and once a person's brain is damaged their life is no longer the same. The purpose of the study was to find out what type of treatment is given to bilingual Hispanics, and what kind of rehabilitation was provided. There are limited studies among bilingual Hispanic people with aphasia. It's not that psychologists, or speech pathologists have not been successful treating bilingual Hispanics, the problem has been treating the bilingual Hispanic patient who has a language disorder. Due to the confidentiality law, the ethnographic study could not be performed. The study was continued using existing data, which was provided by a therapist at an urban facility.

LIST OF FIGURES

Printed in Dunstable, United Kingdom

91222420R00037